PATIENCE
— WITH —
PATIENTS

REVIVING BEDSIDE MANNER

DR. JIM LONGOBARDI, PA, DPM, MBA

LOS ANGELES, CA

Copyright © 2024 by Dr. Jim Longobardi.

All rights reserved. No part of this book may be reproduced in whole or in part without written permission from the publisher or author, except by reviewers who may quote brief excerpts in connection with a review in a newspaper, magazine, or electronic publication; nor may any part of this book be reproduced, stored in a retrieval system, or transmitted in any form or by any means electronic, mechanical, photocopying, recording, or other, without written permission from the publisher or author.

Dr. Jim Longobardi/Patience with Patients
Printed in the United States of America

Although every precaution has been taken to verify the accuracy of the information contained herein, the author and publisher assume no responsibility for any errors or omissions. No liability is assumed for damages that may result from the use of information contained within.

Patience with Patients/ Dr. Jim Longobardi -- 1st ed.

ISBN 9798302563958 Print Edition

CONTENTS

Introduction vii

Chapter 1: The Lost Art of Bedside Manner 1

Chapter 2: The Changing Face of Medicine 9

Chapter 3: People as Patients, not Numbers 21

Chapter 4: The Healing Power of Connection 31

Chapter 5: Bridging the Gap 43

Chapter 6: Empathy Training in Medical Education 55

Chapter 7: The Economics of Compassion 67

Conclusion: Reviving Bedside Manner in Modern Medicine 77

Acknowledgments 83

Author's Bio 85

Dedication

*To my beloved family—Sofie, Emilia, and Gabriella
—who inspire me every day.*

Your unwavering support and love have been the foundation of my journey.

INTRODUCTION

As I look back on my life, I can recall many personal and professional experiences that formed my belief about the importance of "bedside manner," which is the doctor-patient connection built on compassion and empathy.

One stand-out example occurred when I was treating an older female patient. She was suffering from cardiogenic shock, a complication resulting from the inability of the heart to pump blood effectively. This causes the body to shut down peripheral circulation, restricting the flow of blood to your arms and legs in order to increase circulation to your vital organs. As a result, the affected area begins to atrophy and gangrene or sepsis could set in.

In this woman's case, all 10 toes became gangrenous as a complication from the medications used to treat her. The standard procedure would have been to amputate. "Let's just cut off the bad tissue and end the problem."

While this may be an effective and expedient approach at stopping an infection, the loss of a limb can be very demoralizing. For the sake of the patient's mental and emotional well-being, it's best to do what we can to keep their body as whole as possible.

After an examination by her cardiologist, she was referred specifically to me. The cardiologist said, "If there is anyone who can best treat this patient, it is you."

Rather than amputate her entire foot, I decided to remove only the infected part and, working with the cardiologist, do what we could to improve the patient's blood pressure and restore her circulation. Because of our treatment, she still has all of her toes and both feet. For this she is grateful, and her appreciative attitude was a significant factor in her successful recovery.

This example may seem like an obvious decision resulting from the cardiologist and I working together and agreeing on what's best for the patient by keeping in mind her total well-being. But the truth is, such instances are not as routine as they should be. Considering all the additional complications that could have set in, mainly from the patient becoming depressed and not taking care of herself, plus the risk of an excessive use of drugs to ameliorate pain, the outcomes could've been much worse and more expensive.

In working with the patient, in listening to them, in consulting with compassion and empathy, we can greatly improve medical outcomes through this recognition of the importance of a doctor's bedside manner.

CHAPTER 1

THE LOST ART OF BEDSIDE MANNER

Until recent times, a home visit by a doctor was an accepted trope of American life. Such calls represented the distinctive association between a physician and the patient, which led to doctors being regarded as more than medical practitioners, rather as healers with a personal touch that extended far beyond their clinical expertise. Moreover, these intimate and confidential interactions became why the public considered doctors as trusted members of the community. The television show *Marcus Welby, M.D.* exemplified how people wanted to think of their physicians.

The historical significance of bedside manner during this era cannot be overstated—it was a time when medicine was as much about empathy with the patient as it was about diagnosis and treatment.

A Doctor's Presence

During the early to mid-twentieth century, doctors were often deeply embedded in the communities they served. They made house calls, knew their patients by name, and were aware of the intimate details of their lives. The physician's presence was not confined to the examination room, but extended to the very fabric of the community, creating a bond of trust and understanding.

A doctor's opinion carried the weight of education, experience, and wisdom. There were few other professionals who had such a keen and familiar insight into their community and whose pronouncements were so highly esteemed. However, this respect had not been granted but had been earned over decades of proven confidence and close relationships.

Compassionate Care as a Norm

Before continuing, we must define "empathy" and "compassion" as the two words are often interchanged. Empathy means having an awareness and understanding of another's feelings. Compassion is demonstrated through the actions we take in regard to that empathy. Compassionate care is therefore healthcare that takes empathy into account. Empathy and compassionate care are the two necessary components for "bedside manner." If we are to expect positive patient outcomes, then compassionate care must be the norm for healthcare.

The Human Touch

Doctors in the '30s and '40s recognized the therapeutic value of the human touch. Physical examinations were not just clinical procedures, they were opportunities for doctors to better know their patients while conveying warmth and reassurance. This personal connection had a profound impact on patient outcomes by creating profound trust with the medical profession.

While we long for the days of doctor's visits, such house calls are a thing of the past. The reality today is of a much different, and unfortunately, depersonalized, approach to individual healthcare. The bedside manner we promote here is for a more comprehensive appreciation and application of empathy throughout our healthcare provider system. Our goal is for patients to feel valued as individuals, that they've been heard, and that treatments are the result of a physician applying specific and compassionate remedies to their unique conditions.

Given that it would be a rare occurrence for a doctor today to act solely by themselves in treating a patient, we must acknowledge that the doctor-patient connection involves many participants in the healthcare provider system: specialists, nurses, technicians, receptionists.

With so many players in mind, let's discuss who and what contribute to Bedside Manner:

- Foremost is a patient's comfort with their doctor, how their personalities mesh, and how this doctor makes the patient feel.
- Doctor-patient communication is vital if the patient feels that the doctor listens to them and provides clear information about treatment and therapy.
- Trust by the patient for the provider to deliver the skill and quality of care necessary for effective treatment.
- Does the provider's staff interact with compassion and empathy?
- Do visit and wait times take the patient's interests in mind or are they scheduled solely for the convenience of the provider?

Contrasting the Past with the Present

Sadly, medical care by many today is regarded as bothersome treks to a healthcare provider to be examined by electronic devices operated by anonymous technicians, whose priority seems to be processing you as fast as possible as they cycle through a long queue of patients. The warm human touch has been replaced by the hard, cool plastic of an MRI machine with results delivered to you via email.

Previously, a doctor saw you in the familiar comfort of your own home. His or her examination consisted of a hands-on examination during an interview, asking not just about your ailments but also discussing contributing factors that may be affecting your health. Any follow-up examinations—for example, involving x-rays—were conducted by the same doctor who already had a thorough understanding of your medical condition.

Now, your first interaction at the healthcare facility is often a touch screen requesting your insurance number. No wonder you perceive little personal attention, much less empathy with you as a patient. Then you'll be directed to a waiting room, where despite being punctual, you're forced to sit and wait and wait and wait. During this time, you may be asked to fill out a series of questionnaires, many of which you've previously filled out numerous times, giving the impression that your healthcare provider is simply going through the motions of acquiring this information and not paying attention to what they already have.

Next, you'll be ushered by a technician (who has no idea who you are) to an examination room where you wait again. Maybe fill out yet another questionnaire.

When you at last meet your physician, his or her initial move is to pull up your medical chart on a computer screen, rather than acknowledge your presence or ask how you are doing.

The Impact on Patient Well-being

As an appreciation of bedside manner has waned, so too has the overall well-being of patients. A lack of connection with healthcare providers can lead to feelings of isolation, confusion, and mistrust. The shift to a more transactional approach to medicine has left many longing for the days when doctors were not just healers of the body but also nurturers of the soul.

A 2021 study from *The Annals of Family Medicine* reviewed the relationship between a physician's communication style with patients suffering from chronic ailments and their follow-through with medication treatment. The study found that patients who perceived their doctors as more empathetic and compassionate were more likely to adhere to their medication plan, which led to more favorable outcomes such as improved blood pressure and glucose management.

A 2022 report from *Pain Medicine* looked into the interaction between doctor empathy and the pain management of hospitalized patients. Those who expressed receiving greater empathy from their providers reported lower pain scores and more satisfaction with pain management therapy.

Research from 2020 in the *JAMA Network Open* compared surgery recovery with experiences reported by patients. Those who indicated higher satisfaction with their surgeons' communication had better rehabilitation, resulting in shorter hospital stays and lower rates of postoperative complications.

From these examples, we see that years of study into the importance of doctor-patient empathy has shown enormous benefits, not just to patients but to the healthcare industry as a whole. Such an appreciation of a compassionate bedside manner increases patient satisfaction with treatment and encourages adherence to recovery plans. Patients are more likely to follow medical advice when they feel respected, heard, and genuinely cared for by their medical providers.

I've learned that people will forget what you said, people will forget what you did,
but people will never forget how you made them feel.
-Maya Angelou

Feeling acknowledged by their physicians can also lead to better individual mental health outcomes as patients will perceive being supported in their journey to recovery. Compassionate and empathetic communication can reduce a patient's stress and anxiety, as was demonstrated in a study published by the *Journal of Clinical Oncology*.

A positive and empathetic bedside manner can help patients improve personal coping mechanisms and develop better psychological resilience, especially for those in critical care or suffering chronic illness. If we are to encourage the best possible outcomes, a trusting and nurturing bedside manner promoting an open dialogue between doctor and patient is necessary to manifest the benefits of shared decision-making and treatment planning.

And so, here in *The Lost Art of Bedside Manner*, we will journey through time, exploring the roots of compassionate care and examining the factors that led to its decline. By drawing upon the lessons of history, we aim to reignite an appreciation of empathy in modern medicine, rekindling the essence of what it means to truly care for those in need.

CHAPTER 2

THE CHANGING FACE OF MEDICINE

In the relentless march of progress, the face of medicine has transformed, evolving from the noble pursuit of healing to a complex industry shaped by competing interests.

The forces behind the transformation of today's healthcare include the impact of corporatization, the increased workload of physicians and clinical staff, and the prioritization of financial metrics over patient well-being. How has all this change affected the doctor-patient relationship and contributed to the decline of empathy?

The Rise of Corporatization

The metamorphosis of medicine from a personalized, community-driven practice to one managed by vast corporate entities has been a defining feature of contemporary healthcare. Large hospital systems and corporations (pharmaceutical, insurance, private equity) now wield considerable influence over the way modern medicine is administered.

While corporatization does bring benefits: relief for the individual doctor from the hassle of pursuing reimbursements, a standardized quality of care to the patient, and more streamlined coordination with specialists, we have to balance this with its adverse consequences: a greater workload to doctors and clinicians, patients interfacing with the corporation instead of their physician (causing patients to see themselves as numbers in a system), less time spent with individual patients, outcomes driven by corporate metrics instead of what is best for the patient, and less attention focused on delivering compassionate healthcare.[1]

If the single-physician practice was held in such high regard for its bedside manner offering empathy and compassionate care, what then drove doctors from a single-physician practice to one in which he or she is a salaried employee of a corporate healthcare provider? The culprits include the administrative demands of fee payments, confusing regulatory and insurance mandates, the need to contract with outside services such as MRIs and other specialists (and those payment headaches) and rising overhead costs.

As a result of corporatization, by 2021, 75 percent of physicians in the US were salaried employees of healthcare providers. In fact, half of all physician practices are now owned by a corporation. This shift has brought about an increase in healthcare spending, changes in medical practices driven by metrics, and a rise in physician burnout.[2]

Such factors drive individuals out of healthcare altogether, with a shortfall in surgeons predicted for 2036 to be 74 percent of the total needed. The aging population of the US, coupled with declining

---

1. Steven Barrett, "The Corporatization of Primary Care: Unintended Consequences," Perspectives in Primary Care, January 14, 2019, https://info.primarycare.hms.harvard.edu/perspectives/articles/corporatizationofprimarycare.
2. Emily Hutto, "The Cost of Corporatized Medicine, Worse outcomes, increased burnout, and higher costs linked to corporate influence," MEDPAGE TODAY, September 21, 2023, https://www.medpagetoday.com/publichealthpolicy/generalprofessionalissues/106430.

birthrates, means a reduction in available candidates willing to pursue surgery as a career. And consider that today's surgeons are among those professions aging the most into retirement. Fewer available surgeons portend a greater workload for those remaining in healthcare, adding to burnout.[3]

The Insurance Companies

Aside from the healthcare providers themselves, the corporate entities that doctors and patients regard as having the most influence on healthcare are the insurance companies. This perception comes about because when a patient first needs healthcare, the process usually requires approval from the insurer prior to the treatment or service. This prior authorization is intended to make sure the patient receives the care as required by their healthcare plan and that such care is covered by the plan. Unfortunately, the prior authorization process increases workload as it requires that doctors and clinicians navigate cumbersome websites, address changing requirements, provide documentation (often unforeseen), and then wait considerable and inconvenient times for approval.

Other insurer requirements also add expense and time to healthcare, such as Step Therapy, which mandates that physicians have the patient undergo the insurer's treatment protocol instead of relying on the doctor's expertise, especially when referred to a specialist who knows from experience that an MRI is needed and not an x-ray, which just wastes time and money. Insurers may also request

---

3. M. Sophia Newman, "Physician Workforce Data Suggest Epochal Change," *FACS*, American College of Surgeons, 109, Issue 4 (2024), https://www.facs.org/for-medical-professionals/news-publications/news-and-articles/bulletin/2024/april-2024-volume-109-issue-4/physician-workforce-data-suggest-epochal-change/.

additional and substantial documentation to prove the medical necessity for the treatment, and that doctors and the healthcare provider use certain products, whose acquisition benefits the insurer (for example, through a partnership with the product manufacturer). Also, insurers may demand that healthcare providers use specific forms of electronic payment and providers must pay to use those services.[4]

The Pharmaceutical Industry

Another big player in modern healthcare is the pharmaceutical industry, which exists to make money manufacturing and selling drugs. Developing these drugs is timely and expensive, involving years of effort and millions of dollars, with the ultimate goal of a huge payout for the investors.

The challenge for the pharmaceutical industry is that they cannot sell their product directly to the end-consumer—the patient. Notice that TV ads marketing a new drug almost always include the same phrase: "Ask your doctor about…"

The industry relies on doctors to prescribe and make these drugs available. But a doctor cannot receive so much as a pen from a pharmaceutical rep without the risk of accusations that he was influenced by accepting a gift. Which places physicians in a unique position of special trust between the pharmaceutical corporations and patients, who are often grasping desperately at any remedy that promises to reduce their discomfort or suffering.

---

4. Terrence Cunningham, "Five Ways Commercial Insurer Policies Drive Up Costs and Hurt Patients," *American Hospital Association*, May 2, 2022, https://www.aha.org/news/blog/2022-05-02-five-ways-commercial-insurer-policies-drive-costs-and-hurt-patients.

Sadly, given its esteemed position in society, the medical profession has over the decades allowed itself to be corrupted by Big Pharma's big money by participating in rigged clinical trials, publishing favorable articles ghostwritten by the industry, manipulating treatment protocols, and accepting kickbacks. From all this, we see that physicians and healthcare providers have a history of choosing actions based on financial gain over what is in the best interest of the patient.

Another way that pharmaceutical companies can influence healthcare is by partnering with insurers, as we mentioned above, to require the use of products provided by these same pharmaceutical companies.[5]

Private Equity

One aspect of corporatization with a significant influence on the delivery of healthcare involves private equity, which is the ownership of an entity—in this case, a healthcare provider—which is not publicly listed or traded, and generally known as a for-profit-ownership model.

On the plus side, the case for private equity ownership of a hospital is that such a buyout can bring needed capital investment and the financial resources to improve care. However, private equity buyouts tend to target operations that are already doing well financially.

On the negative side, private equity buyouts offload debt on the acquired hospitals, using their assets (buildings, land) as collateral. The acquired hospitals must now generate revenue to pay down the debt, creating incentives, typically cost-cutting measures at the

---

5. Carl Elliot, "Relationships between physicians and Pharma," *National Library of Medicine, Neurology Clinical Practice, 2014 April 4(2): 164-167, https://www.ncbi.nlm.nih.gov/pmc/articles/PMC5765617/.*

expense of the patient. A study of private equity healthcare shows an increase of post-procedure adverse events, such as falls and infection, and a 25 percent increase in hospital-acquired complications with Medicare patients, compared with patients admitted before the private equity acquisition.[6]

Physician Burnout: The Weight of Increased Workload

Physicians today find themselves under the crushing weight of increased workload, which leads to the phenomenon of physician burnout, resulting in emotional exhaustion and a psychological remoteness from patient treatment outcomes. The two major factors for this burnout are increased administrative tasks and productivity pressures.

Increased administrative tasks involve paperwork, insurance documentation, and electronic health records, the latter whose maintenance alone can add an additional nine hours a week on top of the time already devoted to patient care.

Productivity pressures result from the demand for greater efficiency to meet productivity goals, limiting the time doctors spend with a growing list of patients (which can lead to shorter consultations), a diminished connection with patients, and less thorough care.

Other significant factors contributing to physician burnout include difficulties with insurance claims, the rising cost of healthcare, billing issues, and a patient population that keeps getting sicker.

These burnout rates have escalated since 2018, and the adverse results have manifested themselves on healthcare providers and

---

6. Jake Miller, "What Happens When Private Equity Takes Over a Hospital," *Harvard Medical School, News & Research*, December 26, 2023, https://hms.harvard.edu/news/what-happens-when-private-equity-takes-over-hospital.

patients alike. Depression, a disturbing symptom of burnout, has risen in physicians, increasing from 15 percent in 2018 to 23 percent in 2022.[7]

Physician burnout and depression by medical specialties:[8]

- Emergency medicine: 65%
- Internal medicine: 60%
- Pediatrics: 59%
- OB/GYN: 58%
- Infectious diseases: 58%
- Family medicine: 57%
- Neurology: 55%
- Podiatry 31.8%[9]
- Critical care: 55%
- Anesthesiology: 55%
- Pulmonary medicine: 54%
- Oncology: 52%
- Gastroenterology: 52%
- Physical medicine and rehabilitation: 47%
- Surgery, general: 51%
- Diabetes and endocrinology: 51%
- Rheumatology: 50%
- Otolaryngology: 49%
- Allergy and immunology: 49%
- Dermatology: 49%
- Ophthalmology: 48%
- Psychiatry: 47%
- Urology: 47%
- Radiology: 54%
- Plastic surgery: 46%
- Orthopedics: 45%

---

7. Medscape, "Medscape Physician Burnout and Depression Report: Burnout Worsening, Depression Increasing," *PRNewswire*, January 27, 2023, https://www.prnewswire.com/news-releases/medscape-physician-burnout-and-depression-report-burnout-worsening-depression-increasing-301732504.html.

8. Anya Leibovitch, "Physician burnout by specialty: Navigating stress in the healthcare industry," *Tebra: The Intake*, February 23, 2024, https://www.tebra.com/theintake/staffing-solutions/independent-practices/physician-burnout-by-specialty.

9. Daniel R Bonanno, "Burnout in Podiatrists Associated with Individual Characteristics, Workplace and Job Satisfaction," *Journal of Foot and Ankle Research*, 2004 June 17(2), e12003, PMC11080839.

Metrics over Medicine

Seeking ever more efficiency, the healthcare industry has become enamored with metrics—data points that quantify success and guide decision-making. However, this obsession with numbers often results in a skewed prioritization, where financial metrics and productivity take precedence over patient well-being.

A focus on metrics and outcomes can improve aspects of healthcare. Financial metrics allow healthcare staff, patients, insurers, and government regulators to track where and how money is spent. Productivity metrics can provide tools to improve patient care such as treatment checklists, protocols for drugs, and length-of-stay guidelines for hospitalization.

The downside of emphasizing metrics is that it prioritizes specific and measurable outcomes while avoiding a more personalized delivery of healthcare. Doctors are forced to adopt a "check-box" approach to patient treatment, going down a long list of specific questions or concerns to produce a score. Completing this list consumes valuable doctor-patient time, which is already at a premium, and is often done at the expense of doctor-patient communication, necessary to build empathy.

As it's a challenge to measure what is worth measuring, then measures of doubtful utility are monitored in the presumed need to ensure "quality" of care. These measures contribute to a doctor's workload by documenting metrics, such as blood work, eye exams, or vaccinations, which the doctor may feel are not necessary to treat the patient's condition.

Tracking these metrics brings into the healthcare industry yet another layer of staffing that does little to improve patient care while adding more overhead cost and bureaucratic complexity. Such metrics may stem from contracts between hospitals and insurers, in which meeting metric goals could result in reimbursements.

To be sure, reviewing your medical history and medication to provide the metrics of "Med Reconciliation" is a practice lauded by doctors and patients. But would you rather have your physician ask such questions in the sincere act of communicating with you, or that the doctor was simply checking the boxes to pad the hospital's bottom line?[10]

The Technological Paradox

Technology, while a boon to medicine in many ways, has paradoxically contributed to the diminishing appreciation of a doctor's bedside manner. Electronic health records, though streamlining administrative processes, have often transformed doctor-patient interactions into a series of clicks and keystrokes. The many advances of technology have been offset by a myriad of adverse outcomes affecting the healthcare industry and eroding doctor-patient empathy.

Technology can interfere with doctor-patient interactions by reducing direct personal contact. The patient feels more like an anonymous number than a person receiving effective and compassionate care.

Healthcare providers have become more dependent on technology, from the initial interactions with a patient via AI chats on an app replacing human communication, to the use of metrics instead of applying clinical skills to treat patients.

---

10. Victoria R. McElroy, "Why 'Metrics' Overload is Bad Medicine," *National Library of Medicine, Missouri Medicine, 2015 Jan-Feb: 112(1):32-33, https://www.ncbi.nlm.nih.gov/pmc/articles/PMC6170082/*.

Technology brings its unique challenges to the healthcare industry, among them the need for increased vigilance to safeguard data. Electronic health records are prime targets for cyber-attacks to breach access to data or for ransomware. These illegal activities compromise patients' privacy and sensitive medical records, which could lead to identity theft, financial fraud, or lock down a healthcare provider's entire electronic system, denying them the ability to deliver any care at all.

Technology can help prevent some errors, while at the same time, it can introduce new types of worries. Inaccurate data entry, user errors, and system malfunctions could produce billing problems, misdiagnosis of ailments, and unfortunate patient outcomes.

Lastly, technology isn't cheap. The high cost of technology prevents its use for some patients, especially those from low-income neighborhoods. Acquiring, adopting, and maintaining new technology presents significant financial and operational hurdles for even the most advanced and well-funded hospital system.[11]

The Human Cost

Without a doubt, a diminished appreciation of a doctor's bedside manner in healthcare has affected patient treatment outcomes as the personal connection between doctor and patient becomes a casualty of a system driven by financial metrics and the quest for greater efficiency. The irony is that the lack of empathy is actually costing money by complicating patient care and recovery.

The Joint Commission, a US-based global nonprofit that accredits over 20,000 healthcare organizations and programs, studied the

---

11. HM Team, "Is the Effect of Technology on Healthcare Positive or Negative?" HM blog, May 29, 2023, https://verdictvictory.com/blog/effect-technology-healthcare-positive-negative/.

effects of compassionate care upon sentinel events. Compassionate care here is defined as effective communication regarding safety policies, staff communication for handoffs and transitions during patient care, and an understanding of the plan of care.

"A sentinel event" is a patient safety event, not related to the patient's illness or underlying condition, that results in permanent or severe harm, extended healthcare stays, or death. The failure to communicate properly between doctor and patient and among hospital staff, poor teamwork, and not following safety procedures were the leading causes for sentinel events, all evidence of a lack of empathy in patient care. The most common sentinel events in this study were falls while ambulating, falls from beds, and while toileting. Other events include delay in treatment, unintended retention of a foreign object, wrong surgery, and suicide.

The report showed an annual increase in sentinel events, which coincides with the changes to healthcare we've discussed: the corporatization of healthcare, the weight of increased workload, metrics over medicine, and the technological paradox.[12]

As we navigate the changing landscape of medicine, it becomes evident that a course correction is needed. In the subsequent chapters, we will explore avenues to reintroduce compassion, empathy, and patient-centric care into the heart of medical practice, aiming to forge a new path that honors the traditions of healing while embracing the opportunities of modernity.

---

12. The Joint Commission, "Sentinel Event Data 2023 Annual Review," *The Joint Commission*, (2024), https://www.jointcommission.org/-/media/tjc/documents/resources/patient-safety-topics/sentinel-event/2024/2024_sentinel-event-_annual-review_published-2024.pdf.

CHAPTER 3

PATIENTS AS PEOPLE, NOT NUMBERS

In the sterile environment of modern healthcare, the consequences of dehumanizing medical care are palpable, and the toll it takes on a patient's well-being cannot be overstated. In this chapter, we delve into the real-life stories of individuals who have experienced the emotional and physical ramifications of being reduced to mere numbers in the healthcare system.

Neglect in the Emergency Room

Karen's Story: Karen rushed to the emergency room, her pain evident, yet her distress seemingly unnoticed by the staff. Overwhelmed by a high patient load and the pressure to meet time metrics, the medical team failed to address her concerns promptly. The delay in diagnosis and treatment left Karen grappling with a worsened condition, underscoring the importance of timely and attentive care.

Though Karen's experience was an extreme example, it does happen. Emergency rooms, which frequently serve as trauma clinics, often deal with a surge of patients suffering critical life-threatening injuries. You can find children with a dangerously high fever waiting beside mangled car-wreck victims. To physicians, nurses, and medical specialists working in the ER, the pace can be *Boom! Boom! Boom!* They have to triage arrivals, prioritizing attention to those who need immediate life-saving care.

For Karen, the emergency room was her only source of urgent healthcare. While an ER physician did examine her, he found no major problems, only a small ulcer on the bottom of her foot. After reassuring her that it was nothing serious, he asked her to wait for a specialist but in this case, her condition had put her at great risk though the ER physician wasn't aware of this.

Fortunately, I was the specialist on duty in the ER. However, it was after a delay of several hours that Karen was finally assigned to me. Knowing that the ulcer on her foot could be a symptom of a more serious condition, I examined her leg, requested an x-ray, and discovered she suffered from gas gangrene, *clostridial myonecrosis*, a fast-spreading form of gangrene caused by a bacterial infection. Toxins released by the bacteria cause tissue death, which releases gas. The symptoms can develop quickly, and people with a vascular disease such as atherosclerosis or diabetes can experience kidney failure, liver damage, coma, and even death.[13] Treatment such as antibiotics and surgery to remove the dead tissue must be administered without delay. Had Karen gone home without the necessary care, I'm convinced she would not have seen tomorrow.

When patients arrive for treatment in the ER, bedside manner can become an afterthought. Patients are quickly judged and steered to what the medical team decides is most appropriate. With the arrival of so many patients suffering a variety of ailments—burns,

---

13. Ann Pietrangelo, "What is Gas Gangrene?" *Healthline*, July 9, 2017, https://www.healthline.com/health/gas-gangrene

gunshot wounds, poisoning, broken bones—the clinical staff can be dismissive of those whose ailments are not seen as immediately life-threatening, perhaps even trivial.

In my years of practice, I've learned that you must listen to your patients and give them sufficient attention for even simple concerns. I had a patient come into the ER complaining, "My foot's bleeding. It's terrible." I saw that the cut was a very minor injury. Didn't help that he was on meds, which distorted his perception of the situation. But in talking to him, I discovered that his uncle was a diabetic who had cut his foot in a similar fashion, which then got infected, and his leg was subsequently amputated. So, yes, in this patient's eyes, this "little" cut was a big problem.

Misunderstandings in Chronic Illness

Carlos' Journey: Living with a chronic illness, Carlos found himself caught in a web of medical jargon and rushed appointments. The lack of communication and understanding from his healthcare providers left him feeling isolated and defeated. The treatment of Carlos' symptoms did not conform to any readily quantifiable metrics. The emotional toll on his mental health became intricately linked to the management of his physical condition, illustrating the inseparable connection between emotional well-being and health outcomes.

Carlos' example shows what happens as a result of our misunderstandings in the treatment of chronic illness.

The first misunderstanding comes from the perception that a patient needs to look a certain way to be considered "sick." But what is "sick" supposed to look like? Chronic illness can manifest itself in a variety of forms with a variety of symptoms.

And consider when the patient is accused of "faking it" and choosing when to be "sick." A number of variables can affect the patient's condition—changes in the weather, diet, living arrangements, stress—or the patient may just not feel good that particular day.

Patients with chronic illness are told their condition can't be "that bad" because what's driving their symptoms is not readily evident. However, their condition can indeed be "that bad" yet those with chronic illness have no choice but to deal with their ailments. Lifestyle choices are blamed as the reason for the chronic illness when what patients can actually suffer from are genetic autoimmune and autonomic issues, over which they have no control.

After undergoing treatment for chronic illness that has provided little relief, patients can see themselves as burdens to their family and the healthcare system. With this attitude, the patients may give in to despair, which can lead to depression. Physicians have to fine-tune their bedside manner and listen with compassion to those with chronic illness to reassure them that they are no different than anyone else in coping with life's unwanted challenges. Bad things happen to us all.

However, we must be aware that patients may not always be receptive to empathic counsel. If you've been suffering with chronic pain for months, chances are you're not going to be very pleasant. Frustration may cultivate a sour outlook on life, and this will lead to you developing a short temper. Perhaps out of desperation you may say that you're ready to kill yourself if that's what you feel it takes to escape your torment.

For this reason, I never tell my patients there is nothing I can do for them. I lay a hand on their shoulder and say, "I know you're frustrated. We've been looking into this for five, six months, and so far, none of our treatments are working. How do you feel about that? How is your mental health?"

Listen to what they say. You have to read the patient and give them positive feedback. Don't sugarcoat things but do let them appreciate that you take their ailments seriously.[14]

Dismissal of Mental Health Concerns

Kirsten's struggle: Kirsten, a high school student, sought help for her mental health, bravely sharing her struggles with anxiety and depression. Kirsten's deterioration highlighted the repercussions of overlooking mental health and the need for a holistic, patient-centered approach.

In today's focus on mental health, her story is especially relevant. Mental health issues, such as depression, can increase the risk for serious physical health conditions such as diabetes, stroke, and heart disease, and injuries from self-harm.

There are many causes for mental illness. Among the most prevalent are adverse childhood trauma such as child abuse, sexual assault, and growing up in violent environments. Among adults, substance abuse involving alcohol or drugs (or both) can lead to mental illness. Let's not forget environmental factors, such as the effect of social media upon young people.

Those suffering with mental illness harbor feelings of increasing loneliness or isolation. Feeling worthless, they can engage in self-destructive behavior such as substance abuse, high-risk behavior, or self-harm.

---

14. Em + Kate, "The Top 10 Chronic Illness Misconceptions (We're Tired of Hearing)" *Two Being Healthy, Life*, May 7, 2022, https://twobeinghealthy.com/blog/chronic-illness-misconceptions/.

Here in the US, more than one in five live with mental illness, and that includes adolescents. One in 25 adults suffers with a severe mental illness such as major depression, bipolar disorder, or schizophrenia.[15]

Kirsten's health conditions began when several of her classmates starting taunting her, spreading malicious gossip in person and on social media. Though an accomplished athlete, the harassment prompted her to quit the softball team. She managed to keep her grades up, then one day decided to change schools to escape the bullying.

Kirsten's reaction to what she endured is shared by too many of today's youth. Attacks on one's self-esteem, feeling ostracized, FOMO (Fear Of Missing Out) are linked to sleep disruption, memory loss, depression, and poor performance at school. Social media can affect one's physical health even more directly, with anxiety and depression causing muscle tension, joint pain, headaches, and nausea.[16]

Seeking help on how to deal with these problems, Kirsten and her parents attended counseling together. During one session, she related witnessing an argument between her parents. Because of this, the therapist requested a home intervention from Child Protective Services, the visit of which humiliated the parents. During the interview with CPS, they admitted to loud, vocal disagreements but nothing violent. The agent from CPS assured them that all couples had such fights and upon assessing the home situation, left without taking further action.

---

15. CDC Mental Health, "About Mental Health," *CDC Mental Health, Mental Health Basics*, April 16, 2024, https://www.cdc.gov/mentalhealth/learn/index.htm.
16. McLean Hospital, "The Social Dilemma: Social Media and Your Mental Health," McLean Hospital, March 29, 2024, https://www.mcleanhospital.org/essential/it-or-not-social-medias-affecting-your-mental-health.

Her school principals did nothing to stop the bullying, and this episode further eroded Kirsten's confidence in any authority's ability to provide the care she needed. She had also lost respect for the therapist for sending CPS to her home, which could've resulted in her being placed in foster care.

After transferring Kirsten to another school, her parents called the police to report ongoing bullying. However, the police replied that because the incidents occurred in a private school, they could do nothing.

With no relief from the harassment, Kirsten kept spiraling downward. She attempted suicide through an overdose, followed by intensive outpatient therapy. Violent outbursts at the home resulted in calls to the police with one incident having Kirsten taken away in handcuffs. CPS again visited her home, unaware of her history, and so left without doing much more than documenting what they'd seen and assuring Kirsten's mom and dad that they were good parents dealing with trying circumstances.

Kirsten's parents continued to follow through with mental healthcare, doing their best to support her and provide venues for nurturing and positive reinforcement. The path forward was difficult, but Kirsten managed to graduate with honors and proceed on to college.

The experience taught Kirsten and her parents about the challenges of finding compassionate and effective mental healthcare, one with a semblance of a good bedside manner. So-called experts were content to lead Kirsten along, following metrics that did not align with the help she needed. Government bureaucrats were likewise not too concerned that their responses to Kirsten's mental health needs and the contributing causes were not just ineffective, but often counterproductive.

Beyond Physical Ailments

Kirsten's example gives us a lot to think about, starting with her initial visit to therapy. She felt stigmatized by comments about her lifestyle, and because of this interaction, felt that she wasn't being listened to, which she internalized as a lack of respect. In this interaction with authority, her takeaway was judgement, belittlement, and shame. Her reaction was to shut down emotionally, withdraw from others, and refuse to seek care.

Remember that the expectations of patients are different than the expectations of doctors and clinicians. They don't sometimes ask what patients expect from their healthcare. A lot of diagnostics can be deceptively simple, especially for ailments like a cough or a cold: "We'll take good care of you." But when someone's got a chronic, debilitating illness or mental health issues, that takes a lot more patience and understanding than it does to take care of somebody who's coming in for some sniffles. And this treatment can last a long time before you see positive results.

Throughout this process, keep in mind the importance of your bedside manner. You must communicate openly with your patients, with compassion, empathy, and respect. A good bedside manner will yield better patient treatment outcomes, higher patient satisfaction with healthcare, and a greater adherence to treatment plans.

A Call for Change

As we reflect on the stories of Karen, Carlos, and Kirsten, it becomes clear that dehumanizing medical care is not just an inconvenience, it's a critical factor affecting the health and lives of individuals. In the subsequent chapter, we will explore strategies and initiatives for restoring the humanity in healthcare, ensuring that patients are recognized as people, not mere numbers in a system that should prioritize their well-being above all else.

CHAPTER 4

THE HEALING POWER OF CONNECTION

In the ever-evolving landscape of healthcare, one timeless truth remains: the healing power of connection between doctor and patient. In this chapter, we will explore the profound impact of a strong doctor-patient relationship on patient outcomes, drawing on research and studies that illuminate the therapeutic value of empathy, active listening, and personalized care.

The Essence of Healing Relationships
The Patient's Perspective:

Meet Emily, a cancer survivor whose journey was transformed by her oncologist's unwavering support. The empathetic, listening ear provided by her doctor not only alleviated the emotional burden of her diagnosis but also played a pivotal role in her overall well-being.

Emily was diagnosed with breast cancer, which meant years of extensive therapy and anxiety, involving medications and chemo with side effects and complications. What helped ease the devasting news was the doctor's calmness and poise, reassuring Emily that she was in good hands. Besides comforting Emily about the treatment process, the oncologist addressed her other significant worries, particularly regarding family and finances. "How much will this treatment cost? Could I lose my house? If that happens, where would we live? What about the Family Medical Leave Act? Disability? What if I die?"

The Physician's Perspective:

The oncologist, an advocate for patient-centered care, promoted cultivating strong connections with patients. To help soothe the patient, the doctor explained the advancements in cancer treatment. For example, years ago, a diagnosis of melanoma was a death sentence, but it's now more successfully treated. Drugs improving one's immune system have done much to increase the chances for survival. Through shared decision-making with patients and a genuine interest in their stories, the doctor had seen improved treatment adherence and better health outcomes.

Still, when counseling patients about this life-threatening illness, the doctor knew the importance of shepherding them through the five stages of grief: Denial. Anger. Bargaining. Depression. Acceptance.[17]

Upon first hearing that they've been diagnosed with cancer, patients will at first express Denial, saying, "I can beat this. I'm a fighter. I will survive." Then the next day, Anger gives their attitude a 180. "Why me? What did I do to deserve this?"

The oncologist counseled the patient through the remaining steps: Bargaining, Depression (taking special care to avoid the onset of a sentinel event such as self-harm), and Acceptance (making sure that moving forward, the patient takes positive measures).

---

17. Patrick Tyrrell, "Kubler-Ross Stages of Dying and Subsequent Models of Grief," *National Library of Medicine*, StatPearls, February 26, 2023, https://www.ncbi.nlm.nih.gov/books/NBK507885/.

Unfortunately, not all doctors exhibit a constructive and supportive bedside manner. We have this example from an elderly patient being treated for cancer of the white blood cells—myeloma—and who was initially given a prognosis of 10 years. A year later, he saw a different oncologist and after the examination, he asked the doctor, "So what's my prognosis?"

Incredibly, the oncologist replied, "It shouldn't matter to you, you're not going to be here in five months."

Who could ever be this thoughtless and dismissive of a cancer patient's feelings?

From my personal experience, I've overheard versions of the following call from my fellow doctors: "Hello, Mr. Jones, your x-ray doesn't look so good. Might be cancer. Could you come in next week?"

Can you believe delivering such demoralizing news over the phone? But it's something I've witnessed too many times because of the pressure doctors face to regard patients as numbers and not as people. The attitude throughout our healthcare system is *Gotta meet those metrics!*

Empathy as a Healing Tool

In evaluating patient outcomes, we've got to document physiological markers of recovery such as x-rays, blood work, clinical examinations, pain levels, appetites, nausea, and see how these markers are affected by empathy.

In a cohort study of over 1,000 patients treated for chronic lower-back pain, physicians were scored along 10 items according to empathy exhibited during medical encounters.[18] Those doctors rated

---

18. John C. Licciardone, "Physician Empathy and Chronic Pain Outcomes," *JAMA Network*, April 11, 2024, https://jamanetwork.com/journals/jamanetworkopen/fullarticle/2817441.

by their patients as good, very good, or excellent were considered as "very empathic physicians, VEPs," while those with lower scores were "slightly empathic physicians, SEPs."

Patients reported outcomes according to symptoms that included sleep disturbance, pain interference, fatigue, anxiety, and depression. Better outcomes were associated with those doctors with higher scores of patient empathy, showing that bedside manner is an important component of treatment for chronic pain.

While the study noted the importance of encouraging greater physician empathy for those dealing with chronic pain, it also addressed the discourse within the medical community over whether empathy could or should be taught. Some take the position that empathy cannot be measured and so cannot be taught. Others voice that empathy is an innate skill that can be improved with experience. And others advocate that empathy should be integrated into all aspects of healthcare.

Active Listening and Treatment Adherence

Patients who feel heard are more likely to follow through with treatment plans, leading to improved outcomes. Such empathy underscores the importance of moving beyond the transactional nature of medical appointments to foster genuine communication.

A Patient's Perspective:

Meet Julio, an elderly Latino diabetic, who checked in for care after he had hit his foot hard enough to rip the nail of his big toe completely off the nail plate. An examination by a podiatrist determined that because the nail plate was very close to the bone, the injury had to be treated as an open fracture to prevent bone infection.

As the weeks went by, the patient was doing better until the day he came in complaining that his injury had gotten much worse. The color of his toe was dark blue, indicating a lack of oxygen in the tissue with the threat of severe infection. A blood circulation study of his leg and foot did not show favorable results.

Julio was referred to a specialist who performed invasive procedures (such as balloon angioplasties or stents) in his leg to help restore circulation. For the next few days, the doctors had to watch for hyperemia, which is blood rushing back into the affected area, causing the tissue to redden and swell.

The toe no longer looked infected and though scabs started to form, the bone remained exposed. The podiatrist advised, "Unfortunately I think we may get to the point where we may need to amputate your toe. Right now, it's dry, so we're going to leave it alone. If we try to amputate now and with your circulation not being very good, well, we don't want to put the cart before the horse because you may not heal. If that happens, then we might have to go higher, and you may lose your leg. Right now, the best thing to do is to let it dry and keep an eye on it. We'll see you on a regular basis, maybe every week, perhaps get home healthcare visits. Let's take it slow. If you want a second opinion, by all means, get one." The podiatrist also recommended that the patient avoid walking and taking showers. Trips to the bathroom were okay.

The podiatrist noted that his discourse with the patient had become mostly a monologue with little acknowledgment of what had been said. He'd seen that older patients, particularly diabetics, often exhibit a form of dementia.

A week later, Julio and his wife returned. He was livid as the condition of his toe had worsened, and he released a tirade in Spanish swear words against the podiatrist, the clinic staff, and even his wife. Though not fluent in Spanish, the doctor had long served the local Mexican community and so understood most of what was directed at him. He replied that while he realized Julio was upset, it was evident that the patient had not taken care of himself as advised. Furthermore, Julio had to show the doctor and others the same respect he expected in turn.

The podiatrist explained, "I can do my part, but if you don't do yours, then *no bueno*. You can not only lose your leg, but if the infection spreads to your organs, you will die."

Hearing this, the patient began to cry and offered a tearful apology. In the ensuing conversation, the doctor learned that Julio had been frightened by what had happened to him and never thought that the injury to his toe could result in amputation or death.

With that out of the way, the patient agreed to continue seeing this podiatrist and following the treatment plan. Within a few weeks, Julio showed remarkable progress and now his toe is almost back to normal.

This example showed the importance of bedside manner in its various aspects. First, the podiatrist tried to communicate the severity of the injury to the patient and the consequences if treatment was not administered in a timely manner. The doctor also learned through experience the challenge of dealing with older diabetics who may have issues with dementia. When Julio arrived in the clinic overcome with anger, the podiatrist listened, knowing there was more substance prompting the outburst. In his reply, the podiatrist explained the boundaries of expected conduct between himself and the patient. Now that those had been established, they focused the conversation on the importance of following the treatment plan.

Personalized Care and Holistic Health:

We need to study the concept of personalized care and its impact on holistic health. By examining case studies, we can see how tailoring treatment plans to individual needs, preferences, and cultural backgrounds contributes to better patient experiences and outcomes.

A Patient's Perspective:

Meet Karen. She arrived at the clinic with alarmingly discolored toes, and though not a diabetic, her condition was a symptom of a circulatory disease called an ejection infraction, which is the heart not pumping as much as it normally should. If the heart lacks the contractility to perfuse the brain, heart, and other vital organs, then the patient is given vasopressors to increase the blood flow to vital organs. A side effect of vasopressors is to decrease the flow of blood to their extremities. Doing so brings the risk of impaired circulation and infection to the fingers and toes, which this patient had.

The initial consultation to address her condition recommended a partial transmetatarsal amputation: removal of half of her foot. However, the podiatrist offered alternative treatments that could probably save not just her foot, but toes as well. He sat patiently with her, holding her hand as he explained everything they needed to do beyond treatment for her toes such as changes to her nutrition and lifestyle. He included referrals to vascular specialists and a cardiologist. Her treatment included the use of a Vaporox, which contained her foot in a full-oxygen environment with mist therapy. Eventually they were able to stop using the vasopressors and the patient is now on her own with all of her toes.

This holistic treatment contrasts with Step Therapy where the doctors would've had to go through what they considered unnecessary steps before administering the personalized care they knew would ultimately help her. By simply following Step Therapy, the patient might've lost her foot or leg.

Other examples of holistic healthcare include acupuncture, chiropractic therapy, and physical therapy. Mexican barrios have *curanderos*—healers—who attend to the community's healthcare needs. While Western-trained physicians may dismiss many of these approaches, if they make a difference in a patient's well-being, what's the downside?

But as doctors and practitioners of scientific medicine, we must be vigilant in making sure that these treatments lead to the outcomes we're expecting. If the patient has an infection and is drinking some kind of herbal infusion as a remedy, that drink may make them feel better, but it doesn't address the real problem.

Nurturing Connection in Modern Practice
Time as a Healing Resource

We have to address the challenges posed by time constraints in modern medical practice and identify strategies for prioritizing quality over quantity in patient interactions. We must explore innovative approaches, such as extended appointment times or dedicated communication channels, that empower physicians to forge meaningful connections.

One solution to address time constraints is for two practitioners to visit with a patient, assuming both are well-trained, have solid reputations and agreeable personalities, chart well, and interact well with patients and the healthcare staff.

Also, consider having a nurse practitioner, a physician assistant, or another medical technician who can attend to routine tasks and thus free up time for the doctor to focus on the patient.

Another solution involves the practice of *Kaizen*, the Japanese term for continuous improvement. Kaizen became famous as the process the Japanese automobile industry implemented that allowed them to dominate the world car market.

In the healthcare context, Kaizen could mean reviewing activities that are repeated too often, such as data entry or filling out similar forms, and then deciding which steps can be combined and still provide the needed information. In streamlining the process, we must make sure that we haven't eliminated worthwhile redundancies, to avoid situations where the patient may have forgotten to update an important record, like a change in billing address.

For their part, when it comes to change, doctors need to be open-minded. "Just because I've been practicing for thirty-four years doesn't mean I'm not open to new ideas."

A team approach is best. A good boss should train and set up his or her employees for success. Cultivate open communication between specialties, between the staff members, and between departments. People have to be confident that if they identify a problem and propose ways to improve it, someone with "pull" will take them seriously.

Training for Empathy:

Advocate for incorporating empathy training into medical education programs. Highlight successful initiatives that provide healthcare professionals with the skills required to deliver successful outcomes.

When you first meet a patient, it's best to read your audience. If the patient sits there, looking withdrawn, try not to be too sunny and offer a saccharine, "Hi, how are you?"

The patient may be turned off by so much unwanted cheeriness and would prefer a more businesslike approach. The entire visit may go that way, but that is fine. Try to break the ice with questions such as, "How do you wish to be addressed? Do you live close by? Do you enjoy any hobbies? Do you have pets?" Get the patient comfortable talking and that will help lower their anxiety. Perhaps say, "I don't like to feel rushed with my patients. I want to listen and understand what's going on."

But this open approach may not always work. Each patient is different. One might tell you, "I went to a doctor when I was ten years old, and that SOB almost killed me when he stabbed me with this huge injection needle." Even if that never happened, what they remember was a terrible experience.

However, you as the physician need to take charge of the visit and set the tone, striving for a positive encounter focused on the patient's healthcare concerns with commitment to a definitive treatment plan. And never accept the five most dangerous words in medicine: "Maybe it will go away."

A key point that we keep stressing in this book is that establishing empathy with patients improves treatment compliance and outcomes. When patients feel heard as individuals and their concerns are recognized, they will more likely practice self-care and follow their treatment plan. Regrettably, despite all the studies demonstrating the importance of empathy, patients and physicians alike report that much of healthcare still needs to exhibit more empathy.

It is not about the hole in the patient; it's about the whole patient.

Developing a culture of empathy and compassionate care begins at the top, with the leaders of healthcare providers setting the example. For such initiatives to prosper, this culture must be cultivated by instilling an environment where people feel heard and their concerns are taken seriously and acted upon. The rank and file must do their part as well, as building a culture of empathy is the responsibility of everyone involved in healthcare, where each feels appreciated and a useful partner in the treatment process.[19]

Caution: developing empathy cannot be achieved through one training session. Even if metrics show improved patient outcomes after such training, over time, empathy begins to wane as doctors and clinicians return to familiar habits. To maintain and build a culture of empathy requires continuous self-monitoring of emotional connections with patients coupled with updated training. Solicit input from patients and have them contribute to the designing of their healthcare.

A Compelling Case for Change

As we navigate the compelling evidence supporting the healing power of connection, it becomes evident that fostering strong doctor-patient relationships is not just a moral imperative but also a strategic

---

19. Ted A. James, "Building Empathy into the Structure of Health Care," *Harvard Medical School, Trends in Medicine,* January 12, 2023, https://postgraduateeducation.hms.harvard.edu/trends-medicine/building-empathy-structure-health-care.

one. The integration of empathy, active listening, and personalized care into modern medical practice is not only possible but essential for cultivating a healthcare system that prioritizes the well-being of individuals over impersonal metrics. In the upcoming chapters, we explore practical steps and initiatives aimed at reintroducing humanity into the heart of medicine.

CHAPTER 5

BRIDGING THE GAP

As we stand at the gulf between the traditional values of compassionate care and the demands of the contemporary healthcare system, this chapter aims to illuminate practical solutions for closing the gap. By addressing the challenges head-on and advocating for the well-being of both physicians and patients, we can create a bridge that restores humanity in healthcare.[20]

Embracing Technology with Purpose
Streamlining Administrative Burdens:
Administrative burdens are recognized as one of the most significant impediments to efficient healthcare and a major contributor to physician burnout. One remedy would be the streamlining of electronic health record (EHR) systems to allow more time for direct patient interaction, reducing the digital divide between physicians and those seeking care. However, we must monitor technological innovations to ensure that they do not add to administrative burdens instead of easing them.

---

20. Galen Data, "The Disadvantages of Technology in Healthcare," Galen Data, July 27 (2021), https://galendata.com/disadvantages-of-technology-in-healthcare/.

A big aspect of the administrative burden stemming from technology arises from miscommunication between the patient and the healthcare provider. Elderly patients, especially, may not know how to use a computer or phone apps and may also be confused by terminology.

Additionally, apps may be clumsy for older patients to access, particularly those with motor-skill challenges.

Another contributor may be frustration caused by faulty implementation, bringing confusing interfaces or software bugs that require healthcare staff to divert attention away from patients toward fixing the problems. Technology must add efficiency and speed to justify its enormous cost, not introduce obstacles that make more work for everyone.

Yet another contributor to administrative burdens is relying too much on technology. Artificial Intelligence and machine learning can help doctors and clinicians understand and diagnose medical issues, but the risk is that AI modeling may not match real-world circumstances. Doctors may risk becoming complacent and not checking on AI's accuracy as it relates to human medical conditions.

Telemedicine as a Tool, not a Substitute

We need to leverage the potential of telemedicine as a means to enhance accessibility while not glossing over its limitations. The importance of striking a balance, ensuring that technological advancements augment, rather than replace personal connections, is paramount in building empathy between doctors and patients.[21]

---

21. Motti Haimi, "The tragic paradoxical effect of telemedicine on healthcare disparities- a time for redemption: a narrative review," *National Library of Medicine*, BMC *Medical Informatics and Decision Making*, 2023 May 16, V.23(1): 95, https://www.ncbi.nlm.nih.gov/pmc/articles/PMC10186294/.

For many patients, their first experience with telemedicine occurred during the Covid-19 pandemic quarantine. These initial experiences were less than ideal. Internet conferencing platforms such as Zoom were still new and "glitchy," and both patients and providers were trying to figure out how to best share and present information via the screen.

As mentioned previously, elderly patients were the most challenged using telemedicine because of a lack of familiarity with the technology, plus cognitive and physical disabilities.

A significant downside to telehealth remains the challenge of making an accurate diagnosis without being in physical contact with the patient.[22] If the patient needs critical care, the doctor or clinician is under a severe handicap when making a timely and accurate diagnosis. However, doctors can rely on non-medical factors such as a patient's age, gender, location, and information provided by someone other than the patient, such as a parent, to deliver safe care even in pediatric situations.

Other downsides include inconsistent communication with remote or impoverished areas and resistance from communities because of religious or cultural objections to telemedicine.

Since the end of the pandemic, however, we have seen enormous advances in telemedicine. The technology for online meetings has vastly improved thanks to the efforts of Zoom, Google, WhatsApp, and other tech companies. Applications such as Facetime have made people more comfortable communicating via phone video. Also

---

22. Motti Haimi, "The role of non-medical factors in physicians' decision-making process in pediatric telemedicine service," *National Library of Medicine, PubMed, Health Informatics*, 2020 Jun, V26(2): 1152-1176, https://pubmed.ncbi.nlm.nih.gov/31566448/.

consider how many medical devices like electrocardiograms and blood pressure monitors are remotely connected. Smart watches presently detect atrial fibrillation, O2 saturation, and continuous glucose monitoring, and will certainly add more functions to help doctors and healthcare providers keep track of a patient's medical condition in real time.

Meanwhile, you must take into account patients who are very savvy in using the Internet to self-diagnose. A 30-something weekend warrior may come in for a visit and say: "I did a little research online. I'm a runner, I have really good shoes, I run with a club. But now when I step out of bed in the morning, I have heel pain right here. It goes away when I stretch. So I think I have plantar fasciitis, and should I be concerned about anything more serious? What do you recommend?"

In this case, he got the diagnosis just right; 99.9 percent of the time heel pain is caused by plantar fasciitis, but it could be a laundry list of other things. An infection, a torn muscle, a ruptured plantar fascia, even cancer, and so we physicians have to be careful and thorough in our diagnosis, something not possible with telemedicine alone.

Extended Appointment Times and Patient-Centered Scheduling

Redefining Appointment Schedules

We must advocate for a shift in scheduling practices to allow for extended appointment times, which will in turn improve healthcare. This adjustment accommodates the need for thorough communication and fosters an environment where patients feel heard and understood.

A response to the pandemic and the quarantine by patients and doctors alike was the acceptance of the need for online scheduling. This type of scheduling allows providers to leverage technology to improve and simplify healthcare management, increase patient satisfaction, and increase operation efficiency and revenue.[23]

For many patients, one of the most important considerations is the ability to schedule timely appointments. In one survey, 30 percent of patients backed out of an appointment because of long wait times while 20 percent switched doctors because of unreasonable wait times.[24]

Providers can improve patient scheduling by reviewing and revising medical call-center operations, implementing automated responses to patient queries, collecting and analyzing data to identify trends, and incorporating AI to schedule appointments. The use of keywords such as "confirm," "cancel," "reschedule" in automated communication can improve responses by providing intuitive conversational cues. Broadcast messages can improve efficiency by making it easier to quickly reach a large number of patients, especially when sharing similar information such as changing healthcare guidelines.

Patients' familiarity with mobile apps has led to greater reliance on and trust in telemedicine. Patients prefer to receive updates through texts with 95 percent of such messages actually read and responded to within three minutes. This compares with the 16 percent rate of opening email messages. From those encouraging results,

---

23. Artera, "9 Ways to Improve Patient Scheduling – Guidelines and Efficiency," *Artera, Best Practices*, June 29 (2022), https://artera.io/improve-patient-scheduling/.
24. Christopher Rogers, "Prioritizing Online Patient Scheduling Is Imperative In Today's Retail World," *Forbes*, May 17 (2023), https://www.forbes.com/councils/forbestech-council/2023/05/17/prioritizing-online-patient-scheduling-is-imperative-in-todays-retail-world/.

we can see that such mobile app technology can streamline times to schedule visits, update personal information, decrease the number of no-shows, relay lab results, increase patient satisfaction, all of which greatly reduces the healthcare administrative burden.

Allocating Time for Comprehensive Care

We'll discuss the benefits of allocating dedicated time during appointments for addressing the emotional and social aspects of patients' lives. By incorporating a holistic approach to care, physicians can better understand and meet the diverse needs of their patients.

Studies have shown that non-medical emotional and social needs have a profound effect on a patient's health.[25] Even when provided the best available healthcare, if patients have social issues with housing, transportation, safety, and the lack of a strong support system at home (all of which also affect a patient's mental health) then their health outcomes will be far below what's considered ideal. Addressing these social determinants will require a broad holistic approach, the steps of which will be outside the scope of what a healthcare provider may be able to deliver. However, as the most used venue for individual self-care, healthcare providers—as one of the most trusted of all public institutions—are in a unique position to steer public policy to best address how to improve and integrate programs that serve a patient's non-medical emotional and social needs.

---

25. National Academies, "Addressing Patient's Social Needs Within Health Care Delivery is Key to Improving Health Outcomes and Reducing Health Disparities, New Report Says," *National Academies, Sciences Engineering Medicine*, September 25 (2019), https://www.nationalacademies.org/news/2019/09/addressing-patients-social-needs-within-health-care-delivery-is-key-to-improving-health-outcomes-and-reducing-health-disparities-new-report-says.

Recognizing the enormous investment in time, staff resources, and money needed to tackle these social determinants, in the short term, doctors and healthcare providers can acknowledge the impact of social needs upon health outcomes and adjust their care practices accordingly. Alternative medicine and other holistic approaches need to be included in discussions with patients about their healthcare. Physicians can also document health-related disparities regarding social resources and outcomes within their communities.

Long term, doctors and provider staff can help institute data sharing within the healthcare industry and with social service agencies to track how to best direct resources while making the case for more support and funding.

Empathy Training in Continuing Medical Education
Integrating Empathy into Professional Development

Champion the integration of empathy training into continuing medical education programs. By fostering empathy as a core skill, healthcare professionals can enhance their ability to connect with patients on a deeper level, fostering trust and improving outcomes.

Studies into the merits of empathy training have found it effective with many recognized benefits: Patients consider doctor empathy—their bedside manner—an important component of healthcare.[26] Improved patient health outcomes correlate with greater doctor empathy. Empathy allows doctors to better respond to a patient's nonverbal cues during visits, which reduces anxiety and builds trust.

---

26. Christoph M. Paulus, "The effectiveness of empathy training in health care: a meta-analysis of training content and methods," *National Library of Medicine, PubMed Central, International Journal of Medical Education,* 2022 Jan 26, V.13: 1-9, https://www.ncbi.nlm.nih.gov/pmc/articles/PMC8995011/.

This type of connection helps a doctor more fully appreciate their contributions to a patient's health and builds professional satisfaction, which helps reduce burnout.

However, there is a need for doctors to maintain an emotional distance from their patients to better provide an objective analysis for the best care necessary. Balancing this objectivity with patient empathy will lead to the most desired of positive outcomes.

Mentorship and Peer Support

The significance of mentorship and peer support in the medical community cannot be overstated. Creating a culture that values open communication among doctors and provides a supportive network can be instrumental in promoting physician well-being and patient care.

For many successful doctors, a mentor was key to their success in healthcare.[27] Many may assume that in today's electronically hyper-connected world, the idea of a mentor-mentee relationship built through in-person visits may seem outdated, but the truth is, such relationships depend on deep, honest conversations and so are more valuable than those developed in the more convenient and effortless online context.

Mentorships allow for doctors to discuss and weigh career options with a more experienced colleague in their field. These discussions can be with doctors new to medicine or with seasoned veterans who seek advice and counseling to redirect their careers.

---

27. Bonnie Darves, "Physician Mentorship: Why It's Important, and How to Find and Sustain Relationships," *The New England Journal of Medicine, Career Center, February 28 (2018), https://resources.nejmcareercenter.org/article/physician-mentorship-why-its-important-and-how-to-find-and-sustain-relationships/.

Besides mentorship, peer support from work colleagues is crucial to your well-being as a professional.[28] In healthcare, this peer support will be especially significant during periods of high stress, such as during an inquiry about a medical error or for a lawsuit. When this happens, peers and organizations must offer support instead of shame or condemnation.

Peer support can be formal, as from non-mental-health staff within the organization. Informal peer support is when colleagues try to offer support. But this can sometimes be counterproductive because colleagues may feel unsure of what to say or how to help. This is especially poignant as doctors are trained to "fix" a patient's problems, but in these situations, there is little they can do but witness another's trials. For this reason, doctors need peer support training so they can offer constructive encouragement. What must be emphasized is that peer support is not therapy or meant as a substitute if needed.

Physician Self-Care as a Prerequisite for Patient Care
Recognizing Burnout and Stress

The prevalence of burnout and stress among physicians has a serious detrimental impact on healthcare.[29] To address this, we must foster a culture that destigmatizes seeking help for mental health issues and emphasizes the importance of self-care.

---

28. Jo Shapiro, "Peer Support Programs for Physicians: Mitigate the Effects of Emotional Stressors Through Peer Support," *AMA Steps Forward*, June 25, 2020, https://edhub.ama-assn.org/steps-forward/module/2767766.

29. Christine Sinsky, "What is physician burnout?" *AMA Physician Health*, February 16, 2023, https://www.ama-assn.org/practice-management/physician-health/what-physician-burnout#.

The symptoms of physician burnout include emotional exhaustion, a lack of empathy toward patients, and feeling less personal worth. The major factors promoting burnout are not due to personal issues but from the grind of dealing with administrative burdens, system malfunctions, and increased regulatory and technological demands. A 2022 Webinar from the AMA Steps Forward program noted that 52 percent of participants reported a great deal of stress, an increase of 4 percent from the previous benchmark. Fifty-one percent reported burnout, also an increase from the prior benchmark. Burnout affects all specialties and across all healthcare practices.

When doctors experience burnout, the effect on morale and productivity can be considerable. To avoid burnout, staff attention will have to be shifted to administrative tasks at the expense of patient care. Reducing burnout is crucial for maintaining efficient patient care. Solutions for preventing burnout include identifying the factors driving burnout, reducing the causes of stress, and implementing policies and an institutional framework that promote mental and physical well-being.

Balancing Professional and Personal Lives

Advocate for policies that promote work-life balance, recognizing that well-adjusted physicians are better equipped to provide high-quality care. We must pursue initiatives that make physician well-being an integral component of a successful healthcare system.[30]

The medical profession is one of the most demanding of vocations, requiring long hours in high-stress situations that can test a

---

30. Sermo Team, "Guide for doctors: work-life balance best practices," *Sermo*, July 20, 2023, https://www.sermo.com/resources/doctor-work-life-balance/.

doctor's mental and physical health. Achieving a positive work-life balance in spite of the enormous challenges is critical, as this leads to better patient care, increases job satisfaction, and reduces burnout.

Among strategies you can pursue to take charge of your well-being, consider:

Learn to prioritize your responsibilities. However, with so many demands competing for your time and attention, this is easier said than done. At work, identify your most crucial tasks and delegate the less urgent to others. Prioritize time for your personal life and family. Take advantage of technology to help manage your time.

Establish boundaries between your work and personal life. Doctors are by nature Type-A personalities, always ready to take on new challenges. In fact, this attitude encourages physicians to dismiss concerns about their well-being since they make a living solving other people's problems and so believe they know what's best for themselves. But for the sake of your well-being, learn to say no. Try to set limits on work time. Avoid checking work-related texts and emails during your personal hours. Take breaks during the day so you can relax and unwind. Make opportunities to exercise, meditate and enjoy hobbies. Don't hesitate to take vacations.

Probably the most important strategy to deal with the high-stress responsibilities of medicine is to maintain a positive attitude. Acknowledge the satisfaction brought by helping patients and improving the quality of their lives. Practice mindfulness and gratitude. Cultivate a strong support system—family, colleagues, friends from outside work—and use this to maintain a positive mindset, seeking to reduce stress and prevent burnout. To be a good doctor and the best possible contributor to medicine, you must take control of your mental and physical well-being.

A Holistic Approach to Healthcare

By implementing these practical solutions, we can build a bridge that connects the traditional values of compassionate care with the demands of the modern healthcare system. This connection prioritizes the well-being of physicians and patients alike, recognizing that a resilient and supported healthcare workforce is essential for delivering the best possible care. In the subsequent chapters, we will explore real-world examples of institutions successfully implementing these changes and discuss how these practices can be scaled across the broader healthcare landscape.

CHAPTER 6

EMPATHY TRAINING IN MEDICAL EDUCATION

In the pursuit of transforming healthcare into a more compassionate and patient-centered practice, one must start at the very foundation—medical education. In this chapter, we advocate for essential changes in medical education, prioritizing empathy and communication skills. We'll explore successful programs and initiatives that have embraced empathy training, fostering a new generation of healthcare professionals capable of delivering care that extends beyond the clinical realm.

Recognizing the Gap in Current Education
The Missing Link: Empathy and Compassion

We must acknowledge the current gap in medical education, where the focus on clinical expertise often overshadows the development of crucial interpersonal skills. We'll illustrate how this imbalance has contributed to the perceived decline in bedside manner and patient-centered care.

Given how empathy has been shown to improve healthcare, why then is empathy not a priority throughout patient medical care?[31] We've discussed the debate among doctors and clinicians about whether empathy can be taught or measured. What studies have also demonstrated is that among new medical students, there is a strong desire to make empathy central in their approach to improving patient outcomes. At the same time, these students have high and sometimes unrealistic confidence that modern healthcare heals any medical condition. But when students advance into clinical practice, their levels of empathy decline. What happens is that students learn not to listen to their emotions, meaning getting too emotionally invested in a patient, coupled with a curriculum that emphasizes medical knowledge over patient care. So the process of instruction in how to deliver care is itself one major contributor to the decline in empathy. Also, students who scored lower with self-empathy selected specialties with less patient interaction such as radiology or surgery. Not surprisingly, we see that patients report a lack of empathy from healthcare administered by these specialists.

The controversy over whether patient outcomes are best met through care administered using scientific evidence (measurable, repeatable) versus care administered based on intuitive knowledge was examined in a study evaluating the relationships between patients with a chronic disease and their nurses. One contentious detail was how to measure compassionate care.[32] As above in our discussion

---

31. Mohammed O. Razi, "Decline of Empathy among Healthcare Apprentices," *MDPI International Medical Education*, October 5, 2023, https://www.mdpi.com/2813-141X/2/4/22

32. Margreet van der Cingel, "Compassion: The missing link in quality of care," *Science Direct, Nurse Education Today, V. 34, Issue 9 (2014): 1253-1257, https://www.sciencedirect.com/science/article/abs/pii/S0260691714001142?via%3Dihub

of physicians self-selecting specialties according to the levels of empathy likely necessary for that practice, likewise, nurses caring for patients with chronic illness did so believing that more compassionate care (through empathy) would provide for the best outcomes for patients with chronic illness.

The Impact on Patient Outcomes

Let's examine the research showcasing the direct correlation between a healthcare provider's empathetic communication and positive patient outcomes. We shall see that cultivating empathy in medical education is not just a matter of bedside manner but also a fundamental aspect of effective healthcare delivery.

Case Studies of Successful Empathy Training Programs
The Cleveland Clinic Empathy Series:

With the Cleveland Clinic's innovative Empathy Series, we'll examine the results of healthcare professionals engaging in workshops, role-playing, and reflective exercises to enhance their empathetic skills.

One telling example from the Cleveland Clinic Empathy Series podcast followed through on this question from the CEO of the University of Utah Hospital: "How come the patients are mad and the employees are sad?"[33] This prompted a review into their healthcare delivery process, and they discovered that a big part of the issue was that the patient perception of quality care did not match the

---

33. Cleveland Clinic, "The Next Innovation in Experience is High Reliability," *Cleveland Clinic, Studies in Empathy Episodes*, January 1, 2024, https://my.clevelandclinic.org/podcasts/studies-in-empathy/the-next-innovation-in-experience-is-high-reliability.

high care the university thought it was delivering. Their healthcare processes were focused on caregiver convenience instead of the patient. With no other way to share experiences of their healthcare, patients turned to public and third-party review sites, where the preponderance of reviews was negative. While the hospital thought they were delivering first-class quality healthcare (which they probably were), public comments did not support that. However, by soliciting feedback directly from patients, this provided a mechanism in which they felt invested in a relationship with a provider who did value their opinion. This process added transparency since doctors could make correlations to specific patients, their conditions, and the outcomes, and so adjust their practices accordingly.

Despite this appreciation for patient engagement, the initiative discovered that patients were not always eager to provide feedback. When patients were deeply concerned with their outcomes, the engagement levels were high. Otherwise, the engagement level was low, and this was attributed to the patients trusting the care they were receiving. The initiative found not that they need to teach doctors and providers to care more, but that they should focus on structures and processes that build relationships with the patient and communicate healthcare treatments that the patient will follow.

Which aligns with our premise about the importance of empathy—of bedside manner—by having the patient believe they are in a caring relationship with their doctor (and not simply a number in the system) and that their concerns are heard and addressed.

Another example from the Cleveland Clinic Empathy Series demonstrated how compassionate healthcare can deliver positive health outcomes even with a troublesome patient.[34] In this case, he was a middle-aged smoker, with a history of cancer and coronary heart disease. He harbored a distrust of the medical system and aggressively questioned his diagnosis and treatment.

This doctor took him on as a new patient and decided to sit with him and his wife to listen to their concerns. Turns out, the patient had a bad experience with his previous healthcare. The doctor knew she had to build trust with him, make him feel valued and listened to. After their consultation, she developed a treatment plan and scheduled an echocardiogram. The results showed disturbing abnormalities, requiring urgent care, and the doctor went looking for the patient. In the meantime, he had disappeared. Fortunately, the doctor tracked him down before he left the hospital and was able to convince him to remain and get the care he needed. The patient replied that he wouldn't have listened to anyone but her, affirming the connection she had made with him. Making the extra effort to understand him as a human being and not simply a number on a chart was what had secured his trust in her.

To show the value of a personal connection between caregiver and patient, this podcast related that when a patient's photo is attached to radiology results (in essence putting a face to the chart), the results become more accurate. This illustrates the power of compassionate care: when you see patients as people and not just numbers, then providers give better care.

---

34. Cleveland Clinic, "Tales from a Resident," *Cleveland Clinic, Studies in Empathy,* November 1, 2023, https://my.clevelandclinic.org/podcasts/studies-in-empathy/tales-from-a-resident.

The Jefferson Scale of Empathy:

Among the most significant tools implemented to develop empathy in medical schools is the Jefferson Scale of Empathy, which provides metrics for assessing and promoting empathy among medical students.[35] Several leading healthcare teaching institutions have integrated this tool into their curriculum, fostering a culture of empathy from the beginning of a student's medical education.

The Jefferson Scale of Empathy was developed as part of a nationwide Project in Osteopathic Medical Education and Empathy, sponsored by the American Association of Colleges of Osteopathic Medicine, American Osteopathic Association, and the Cleveland Clinic. The study sought to define and measure "empathy" and to determine how to use empathy to improve patient outcomes. As mentioned previously in this book, while empathy is regarded as a significant component of healthcare, there exists debate about what is "empathy" and so how to teach it, if that is even possible.

The project defined empathy in regard to patient care as "predominantly cognitive," involving an "understanding" of the discomfort and pain, with "a capacity to communicate this understanding," coupled with "an intention to help."

A national norm table for the assessment of the JSE was developed from a sampling of first-year students at US colleges of osteopathic medicine. These JSE metrics have since been used to score medical students, healthcare practitioners, and health professional

---

35. Mohammadreza Hojat, "The Jefferson Scale of Empathy: a nationwide study of measurement properties, underlying components, latent variable structure, and national norms in medical students," National Library of Medicine Adv Health Sci Educ Theory Pract. 2018 Dec;23(5):899-920. https://www.ncbi.nlm.nih.gov/pmc/articles/PMC6245107/

students who are not medical students. JSE items used for the 20 item-score correlations included: Place of emotion in medical treatment, Nonverbal cues and body language in understanding patients, with these grouped into the three latent variables of Perspective Taking, Compassionate Care, and Walking in Patient's Shoes.

The study found that women received higher JSE scores than male participants, ascribed to gender differences in expressing empathy, social learning, genetics, and evolutionary development.

In keeping with findings from other initiatives, the JSE study found that medical students and physicians choosing "people-oriented" specialties (general internal medicine, family medicine, pediatrics, and psychiatry) obtained higher JSE scores than those in "procedure-oriented" practices such as surgery, pathology, radiology, anesthesiology, and urology. From this, we can see that students perceived as having more empathy self-select for specialties where they have more direct-patient interaction, and students perceived as having less empathy chose specialties where patient contact is more procedural or technology based.

Whether empathy actually translated into improved patient outcomes was analyzed in a study of diabetic patients, with lower rates of hospitalizations recorded for patients of doctors with higher JSE scores.

Incorporating Empathy Training into the Curriculum
Integrating Communication Skills Courses

Advocate for the integration of communication skills within the medical curriculum. We need to emphasize the importance of teaching active listening, effective communication, and compassionate bedside manner as core components of medical training.

A study published by the National Library of Medicine explored medical students' empathetic communication skills in clinical practice.[36] Students observed clinicians' behavior during interactions with patients and noted that clinicians who demonstrated empathetic communication skills, an awareness of a patient's body language, and addressed a patient's healthcare needs, were better able to improve the management of the patient's outcomes. Conversely, clinicians who limited their time during interactions with patients and who seemed to lose "mental energy," saw a diminished awareness for the patient's condition.

Student takeaways from the study included: the recognition of empathy; a greater appreciation of empathy and its positive influence on patient healthcare outcomes; and that empathy can be learned and those communications skills improved upon.

Real-World Clinical Simulation:

Now we'll look at the use of realistic clinical simulations that incorporated empathy training and discuss the results of a medical school that utilized simulated patient encounters to provide students with practical experiences in navigating the emotional and interpersonal aspects of healthcare.

In the ongoing effort to integrate empathy into healthcare practice, one study from a Chinese Neonatal Intensive Care Unit (NICU) used simulation-based training to improve the communication skills

---

36. Elize Archer, Ilse S. Meyer, "Applying empathic communication skills in clinical practice: Medical students' experiences," *National Library of Medicine, South African Family Practice, 2021 Feb 9, 63(1):e1-e5.* https://www.ncbi.nlm.nih.gov/pmc/articles/PMC8378147/.

of neonatal nurses.[37] Given the lack of a conclusive definition of "empathy," this study decided upon an understanding and appreciation of another person's feelings and being able communicate that understanding back to the patient.

Thirty-two nurses from the NICU were selected for the three-month course of instruction taught by a nursing psychologist, a pediatrics specialist, and two head nurses from the NICU. At the end of the training, over 93 percent of the nurses self-reported that they were satisfied with their ability to better recognize empathy, assess behaviors in clinical settings as they affected patient outcomes, and so improve their communication skills.

However, as the training was in simulated conditions, more work was needed to analyze how these nurses could apply in actual clinical settings what they had learned.

Building a Culture of Empathy in Medical Schools Faculty Development Programs:

Let's highlight the significance of faculty development programs that can equip educators with tools to model and teach empathy. What institutions have successfully implemented initiatives that fostered empathy in both faculty and students?

Can Medical Schools Teach Empathy?

The evidence cited thus far shows that increased levels of empathy improve patient healthcare outcomes. Empathy allows a physician

---

[37]. Yu Na Shao, "Simulation-Based Empathy Training Improves the Communication Skills of Neonatal Nurses," *Science Direct, Clinical Simulation in Nursing, V. 22:* 32-42, September 2018, https://www.sciencedirect.com/science/article/abs/pii/S1876139918300537.

to better understand and diagnose their patients and so deliver more effective patient-centered medical care. Despite this benefit, it's been shown that empathy decreases during medical education, and that part of the problem is that there is no extensive curriculum to teach empathy.[38]

The reason for this decline in empathy is the opinion that medical care can only be taught in controlled settings where students observe physicians who practice medicine without the need for empathy. Without including empathy into the formal curriculum, it's no surprise that students learn to value efficiency over understanding.

Some practitioners propose medical training similar to that of a physical examination, incorporating explicit instruction, teaching in clinical settings, and the critical observation of resident physicians, with emphasis on learning through repetition. As physical examinations allow for the objective assessment of a student's interaction with real patients, such a practice should also include demonstrating empathy and compassionate communication skills.

Simulations can be included within the curriculum in clinical settings to best teach empathy, providing for standardization and reproducibility. Role-playing both the physician and patient will help a student gain an appreciation of the communication needed during a medical interaction.

Students would be scored according to the Jefferson Scale of Patient's Perceptions of Physician Empathy. Those with low scores would not be penalized but instead counseled on how to improve their empathic skills while still in medical school. Physicians who

---

38. Kostantinos E. Morris, "Creating a Medical School Curriculum to Teach Empathy," *National Library of Medicine, Annals of Surgery Open, 2021 Aug 5, 2(3):e085,* https://www.ncbi.nlm.nih.gov/pmc/articles/PMC10455068/.

exhibit model empathetic skills would be selected for clinical rotations. The goal of this proposal is to teach a cohort of physicians who can better understand their patients and so improve outcomes. Long-term objectives would be for medical teaching institutions to help quantify empathy and promote its inclusion into the curriculum.

Student-led Empathy Initiatives:

We need to celebrate the impact of student-led initiatives advocating for empathy in medical education. We'll look at one example of a student-driven program that raised awareness for empathy and promoted a culture of empathy within the medical school community.

A student-led study by the University of Iowa Internal Medicine Residency Program examined empathy at several of the university's health colleges, among them the Carver College of Medicine and the colleges of Pharmacy, Dentistry and Nursing.[39] The study of 300 students concluded that their empathy score was associated with their perception of faculty members' empathy to patients (and students).

The study showed that teachers must lead by example by modeling empathetic behavior in the learning environment. Among the skills learned: a strengthened sense of self-awareness, to discern progress in developing empathy, and good personal behavioral practices such as the value of eye contact, asking open-ended questions, avoiding interrupting the other person, and confirming an understanding of what was shared.

Feedback opportunities with instructors provided students time to reflect upon and learn from their experiences.

---

39. Trevor Jackson, "Can Medical Schools Teach Empathy?" *Medicine Iowa, Fall 2023*, https://medicineiowa.org/fall-2023/can-medical-schools-teach-empathy#.

The Future of Medicine: Empathetic Healers

As we advocate for these changes in medical education, it becomes clear that the future of medicine lies in the hands of empathetic healers. By prioritizing empathy and communication skills in medical education, we can ensure that the next generation of healthcare professionals is equipped not only with clinical expertise but also with the ability to forge deep connections with their patients, ultimately redefining the landscape of healthcare. In the following chapter, we will delve into how these empathetic practices can be integrated into the broader healthcare system.

CHAPTER 7

THE ECONOMICS OF COMPASSION

In a healthcare landscape often dominated by financial considerations, there exists a pervasive notion that profit and compassionate care are mutually exclusive. In this chapter, we challenge this assumption, exploring examples of healthcare systems that have successfully integrated both economic viability and compassionate care. By highlighting these examples, we aim to underscore the long-term benefits for patients, providers, and the healthcare industry as a whole.

Dispelling the Myth: Profit vs. Compassion

The Perceived Dilemma:

We need to challenge the prevailing belief that prioritizing compassion in healthcare jeopardizes financial sustainability. We'll delve into the historical context that has perpetuated this dichotomy and examine its impact on patient care.

The True Intersection:

Are profit and compassion inherently contradictory? Let's explore the potential intersection where economic viability and compassionate care not only coexist but mutually reinforce each other for the benefit of all stakeholders.

Economic viability and compassionate care can benefit each other through an approach called value-care—which positions patient outcomes with financial incentives.[40] Value-care encourages collaboration among healthcare providers and the medical industry to improve patient outcomes by shifting attention from treating symptoms to a holistic approach addressing all aspects of a patient's well-being. One value-care initiative to accomplish this leverages technology and data collection to facilitate patient interaction—which includes telehealth—that leads to determining patterns, quantifying outcomes, and accumulating that data for decision-making.

To successfully implement value-care will require the buy-in from healthcare provider leadership. Previously, stakeholders—physicians, clinicians, administrative staff, educators, industry, insurance, regulators—often worked in silos and now they must collaborate on delivering patient-centered healthcare.

To enhance economic viability, one objective of value-care will be to incentivize preventive care and early interventions. This can be achieved by reducing barriers to healthcare such as extended wait times or the availability of limited resources. By quantifying financial expenditures to healthcare outcomes, this process can provide metrics to help streamline healthcare and reduce costs.

By making value-care the central approach to delivering healthcare, patient-centered care will be both more compassionate and profitable.

---

40. Integrity Billing, "Unleashing Profits and Compassion: How Value-based Care Revolutionizes Behavioral Health," Integrity Billing, January 12, 2024, https://integritybillingco.com/blog/unleashing-profits-value-based-care/.

Successful Integration of Compassion in Healthcare Systems

The Mayo Clinic Model:

Explore the Mayo Clinic's renowned patient-centered care model, emphasizing the institution's commitment to compassionate care alongside its financial success. Showcase how the Mayo Clinic's emphasis on patient satisfaction and positive outcomes has contributed to its long-standing reputation and financial stability.

Without a doubt, when discussing patient-centered care, the Mayo Clinic is usually what first comes to mind because it consistently ranks above other healthcare providers.[41] This reputation arises from the clinic's core value of putting the needs of the patient first. To further advance this priority on quality care, the Mayo Clinic developed a covenant that more fully articulated its principles through the Mayo Clinic Model of Care and the Mayo Clinic Model of Education.

From its beginning in the early 1900s, the Mayo Clinic has devoted its efforts as an institution to encourage the education and development of doctors, clinicians, and healthcare staff to meet the highest standards of professionalism regarding individualized patient care.

The Mayo Clinic's medical staff and students pursue excellence as measured by healthcare results achieved through collaboration in mandated and voluntary initiatives, the goal of which is continuous improvement and better patient outcomes. Furthermore, the clinic

---

41. Thomas R. Viggiano, "Putting the needs of the patient first: Mayo Clinic's core value, institutional culture, and professional covenant," National Library of Medicine, Academic Medicine, 2007 Nov, 82(11):1089-93, https://pubmed.ncbi.nlm.nih.gov/17971697/

has been at the forefront of the digital transformation of healthcare with its Clinical Data Analytics Platform that takes advantage of AI and machine learning.[42]

Kaiser Permanente's Preventive Care Approach:

We'll now turn our attention to Kaiser Permanente and its focus on preventative care and patient education, showcasing how an investment in compassionate, proactive healthcare can lead to reduced long-term costs.[43] This approach not only manifests a positive impact on patient outcomes but can also contribute to the financial sustainability of healthcare organizations.

An industry leader known for delivering quality, patient-centered healthcare, Kaiser Permanente emphasizes that its actual work as a healthcare provider is not about clinics, or surgical centers, or research laboratories, or maintaining hospitals, but about the importance of a doctor's bedside manner when interacting with a patient.

To follow through with this philosophy, Kaiser Permanente leans on team-based care and uses evidence-based processes gathered from its innovative electronic records system. As one of the nation's largest healthcare providers, Kaiser Permanente has the capital resources to maintain a research infrastructure, allowing them to develop and implement innovations within about 26 months compared to the industry-wide standard of 17 years.

---

42. Jay Furst, "Mayo Clinic's patient-centered values and culture drive its 2030 strategy to cure, connect and transform health care," *Mayo Clinic News Network*, February 25, 2020, https://newsnetwork.mayoclinic.org/discussion/mayo-clinics-patient-centered-values-and-culture-drive-its-2030-strategy-to-cure-connect-and-transform-health-care/.

43. Vincent J. Felitti, "Kaiser Permanente Institutes of Preventive Medicine," *National Library of Medicine, The Permanent Journal*, 2004 Winter; 8(1):3-5, https://www.ncbi.nlm.nih.gov/pmc/articles/PMC4690702/.

Knowing that its people are ultimately the key to success, Kaiser Permanente strives to maximize the potential, the creativity, and the abilities of its extensive healthcare workforce.[44]

Accountable Care Organizations (ACOs):

Let's analyze another venue offering value-care by reviewing the experience of Accountable Care Organizations, whose business model is to prioritize patient well-being using care coordination. These ACOs have not only improved patient outcomes but have also realized financial profits through reduced hospitalizations and better management of chronic conditions.

An Accountable Care Organization (ACO) is a group of doctors, hospitals, and other care providers such as specialists and clinics, and in some instances, insurance companies, voluntarily working together with the goal of providing high-quality patient healthcare at reduced costs. The participants seek to maximize healthcare by incentivizing controlled costs by avoiding unnecessary procedures and tests.[45]

For example, in a traditional fee-for-service system, such as Medicare, doctors and healthcare providers are paid for every procedure and test performed. With an ACO, providers are rewarded if they perform fewer procedures that produce better outcomes. With this approach, physicians and providers must satisfy specific standards of care centered on prevention, quality care, and improved

---

44. Kaiser Permanente, "World-class care proven to deliver exceptional outcomes," *Kaiser Permanente, Business*, 2024, https://business.kaiserpermanente.org/kp-care-value/exceptional-care.

45. Med USA, "The Pros and Cons of Accountable Care Organizations," *Med USA, Practice, Group Management Tips*, June 24, 2020, https://medusarcm.com/blog/pros-and-cons-of-acos/.

outcomes. Payment is based on quality of results instead of quantity of services. In this collaborative approach, providers can review a patient's tests and procedures to avoid unnecessary work.

But an ACO does have drawbacks. Among them, participating in an ACO could require extensive reorganization of the practice's business model, and such costs may be prohibitive for smaller providers. An ACO would also require investment in digital software, hardware, and the accompanying support staff. Additionally, if an ACO cannot meet its performance objectives, or if its healthcare processes do not result in savings, then the participants could expect to pay penalties.

The Long-Term Benefits for Patients, Providers, and the Industry

Improved Patient Satisfaction and Outcomes

Let's review the evidence demonstrating that compassionate care contributes to higher patient satisfaction and improved health outcomes. We'll look at the long-term benefits of a satisfied patient population, including loyalty and positive word-of-mouth referrals.

The value of compassionate care has been long studied and the consensus is that for the patient, compassionate care improves the following of treatment plans, promotes healing, and enhances both physical and emotional well-being.[46] For physicians, the benefits include less burnout and depression, a greater sense of purpose, and more diligent patient care. Healthcare providers also benefit, as it

---

46. Stephen G. Post, "Compassionate Care enhancement: benefits and outcomes," *The International Journal of Person Centered Medicine*, September 22, 2011, https://www.stonybrook.edu/commcms/bioethics/_pdf/CCE.pdf.

enhances their reputation for delivering quality care with a more cost-effective use of resources and time while reducing exposure to malpractice lawsuits.

When patients feel better connected to the physicians, and more emotionally at ease, they are more likely to follow treatment plans, which in turn improves outcomes. Taking into account that 30 percent of every dollar spent on healthcare is the result of a patient not following treatment plans or from poor self-care, then the investment in a compassionate approach to healthcare will yield positive dividends.

A culture of compassionate care—of a good bedside manner—throughout the healthcare establishment from medical school, through residencies, in clinics, and among staff will improve the financial "bottom line" by reducing the costs of patient care, improving physician well-being and their focus on work, streamlining provider services, and lowering the risk of expensive malpractice lawsuits.

Another significant gain from compassionate care comes from the favorable word-of-mouth referrals from satisfied patients and their families. More than any other means of marketing a healthcare practice, positive and trusted word-of-mouth reviews and referrals bring the most benefit to a provider's credibility and profitability.[47]

Physician Well-being and Retention:

In discussing how a culture of compassion contributes to improved physician well-being and job satisfaction, we'll explore examples of

---

47. Lauren Parr, "How To Get More Word-of-Mouth Patient Referrals in a Digital World," Forbes Communication Council, October 8, 2020, https://www.forbes.com/councils/forbescommunicationscouncil/2020/10/08/how-to-get-more-word-of-mouth-patient-referrals-in-a-digital-world/.

healthcare organizations that have successfully retained talented healthcare professionals by prioritizing their sense of purpose and fulfillment.

One medical specialty known for its high rates of burnout and low retention is that of emergency physicians. However, it is possible to buck this trend and one provider, SouthlandMD, demonstrated how its efforts brought it distinction as one of the top employers for emergency medicine.[48] To reduce burnout and turnover, SouthlandMD emphasized open communication between doctors and patients, doctors and staff, a focus on work-life balance, and educational opportunities for its emergency physicians. But key to SouthlandMD's approach to physician retention and fostering an enriching work environment was its acknowledgment that when doctors feel appreciated and supported in their efforts to make a positive difference in patient outcomes, in other words, emphasizing compassionate care, then physicians, patients, and the provider all benefit.

Enhanced Reputation and Community Trust:

One of the intangible yet invaluable benefits of compassionate care is how it will enhance the reputation of a healthcare provider with the community and improve trust. Healthcare organizations with a reputation for compassionate care attract philanthropic support and cultivate community engagement.[49]

---

48. SouthlandMD, "SouthlandMD Ranks #1 for Highest Overall Retention Among Emergency Physicians in the Country," *SouthlandMD*, March 15, 2024, https://southlandmd.com/press_releases/southlandmd-ranks-1-for-highest-overall-retention-among-emergency-physicians-in-the-country-by-em-news/.

49. Émilie Lessard, "How does community engagement evolve in different compassionate community contexts? A longitudinal comparative ethnographic research protocol," Sage Journals, Palliative Care and Social Practice, 2023, V. 17, https://journals.sagepub.com/doi/full/10.1177/26323524231168426.

Community engagement is one crucial component of healthcare for those suffering a complex, serious, and sometimes terminal illness. However, this community engagement has not been adequately studied to determine how to best align resources to assure the necessary quality of care. Such research could provide information by analyzing community engagement among its constituents, bringing in the broad scope of societal factors and the resultant effect on health outcomes.

One major player in this community engagement is healthcare philanthropy.[50] This aspect of philanthropy focuses on the raising of funds to support healthcare organizations in the promotion of their mission and outreach. The use of these funds ranges from providing financial assistance for patients to promoting awareness for healthcare causes to supporting medical research.

Philanthropy depends on community engagement to both raise awareness for the causes it supports and to cultivate a sense of collaboration within that community. For those involved in philanthropy either as donors or as professionals, they seek to make a positive difference in people's lives, with that sense of accomplishment amplified by the satisfaction knowing that their financial investment will ultimately improve healthcare and save lives.

A Call to Action: Integrating Compassion and Economics

We must challenge the healthcare industry to reconsider its priorities, emphasizing that the integration of compassion is not only morally right but also economically sound. Encourage policymakers,

---

50. Association for Healthcare Philanthropy, "My Purposeful Path: Why you should consider a career in healthcare philanthropy," Association for Healthcare Philanthropy, 2024, https://www.ahp.org/mypath#.

healthcare leaders, and professionals to explore and adopt models that showcase the viability of compassionate care within a financially sustainable framework. As we move forward, the challenge lies not in reconciling profit and compassion but in recognizing that the two can be powerful allies, shaping a healthcare landscape that prioritizes the well-being of all its participants. In the Conclusion, we'll explore practical strategies for implementing this paradigm shift in healthcare organizations of all sizes and structures.

CONCLUSION

REVIVING BEDSIDE MANNER IN MODERN MEDICINE

As we wrap up this exploration into the evolution of healthcare, from the compassionate doctors of the 1930s and '40s to the complex and demanding landscape of modern medicine, one resounding truth emerges—the crucial importance of reviving bedside manner. The art of compassionate care, once the heartbeat of healing, has suffered erosion over the decades, leaving patients yearning for the personal touch that was once a hallmark of medical practice.

In this journey through time, we witnessed the transformation of medicine from a community-driven, empathetic practice to a fast-paced, profit-oriented industry. The consequences of this shift are evident in the stories of patients who have felt neglected, misunderstood, and dismissed—a stark contrast to the compassionate care offered by doctors in the past.

It is time for a call to collective action, a rallying cry to reshape the culture of medical care. Healthcare professionals, institutions, and patients must join forces to place empathy, understanding, and the patient's well-being at the forefront of our healthcare priorities. By recognizing the intrinsic value of a strong doctor-patient relationship, we can work towards reintegrating the human touch into modern medical practice.

We've seen a lot of strides toward improving healthcare by using telehealth, teleradiology, and telecardiology. Communication between providers and patients has advanced through the use of apps, for example, that allow for more timely contact between doctors and providers and patients for scheduling and for sharing test results.

On the other hand, progress is offset by a growing medical bureaucracy and increasing government regulation, all of which adds expense and more demands to a physician's already oppressive administrative burden. Inflation also contributes significantly to rising healthcare costs. And all that wonderful new technology doesn't come cheap, and neither does the expertise needed to implement and maintain it.

Additionally, we have systems in place, such as state-funded insurance, that traditionally reimburse low rates for a physician in private practice, making it difficult for them to provide quality care. However, a Federally Qualified Health Center (FQHC) gets $200, making treating the patient worth their time. FQHCs may see up to 70 of these patients a day, which adds up to a lucrative sum. And what patients they don't see get farmed to the emergency room.

The downsides for a private practice to join an FQHC are the increased volume of patients and that there are few incentives for preventative healthcare, meaning you tend to see patients with complex and expensive medical conditions.

Another factor affecting compassionate care is the volume of work that doctors must shoulder. The fewer doctors available, the heavier the burden that now must be distributed among the remaining physicians. Unfortunately, the number of people finishing medical school isn't keeping up with demand and especially the needs of an aging population. By 2035, we're going to see a huge drop in the number of surgeons with a corresponding increase in workload on the remaining specialists.

Moving Forward:

In the previous chapters we've related many examples of studies showing that empathy and compassionate care improve patient outcomes, reduce physician burnout, and increase the efficiency of healthcare. To emphasize the effect of compassionate care on patient outcomes, a study cited by Stanford Medicine showed these benefits: improved blood-sugar control among diabetic patients; that on average, medical costs fell by 50 percent; and a faster recovery of symptoms with fewer referrals, tests, and visits.

There remains much debate about how to measure empathy, whether it is an innate trait or a skill that can be acquired, and therefore, is it even possible to quantify compassionate care?[51] However, takeaways of physician-patient interactions have identified four specific behaviors that physicians (and clinicians) can exhibit to express compassion in the form of bedside manner:

- If the patient is bedridden or sitting, you should also sit instead of standing when speaking with them.
- Use face-to-face contact with eye contact. A challenge of course if using telehealth.
- Show an interest in the patient's emotional and psychological well-being.
- Don't interrupt.

---

51. Stanford Medicine, "Compassion: A Powerful Tool for Improving Patient Outcomes," *Stanford Medicine 25, An Initiative of the Program for Bedside Medicine*, 2024, https://stanfordmedicine25.stanford.edu/blog/archive/2019/compassionimprovingoutcomes.html.

Another initiative that uses empathy to expand compassionate care is that of Narrative Medicine, which is when physicians and clinicians connect with writers, artists, academics, and chaplains in a collaborative effort to document a patient's life story as it relates to their medical condition.[52] This can be an especially powerful tool to help patients dealing with chronic pain, intensive long-term therapy, or severe trauma. The stories collected with narrative medicine can be shared as videos, in magazines and anthologies, or in podcasts. This approach helps healthcare providers, and the public, better understand and improve medicine from the experiences of patients and physicians.

Since we know that a major cause of burnout and the deterioration of bedside manner is the volume of patients and the workload demanded of a doctor, aggravated by a growing shortage of doctors, we need to incentivize our economy to encourage more people to become doctors. As the expected cost of a medical degree is around half a million dollars in the form of student debt, that alone is enough to discourage many candidates. However, simply providing subsidies to pay for medical education is not enough. Whatever programs are established to help pay for a medical degree must be accompanied by a requirement for the individual to give back to the community.

Our Electronic Future:

As the use of AI in healthcare continues to accelerate, we need to be cautious not to over-sell its utility or place in healthcare, especially when it comes to situations requiring empathy and compassionate

---

52. Columbia University, "Division of Narrative Medicine," Columbia University Department of Medical Humanities and Ethics, 2024, https://www.mhe.cuimc.columbia.edu/division-narrative-medicine.

care.[53] We note with AI that face-to-face personal contact, a critical component of compassionate care, is absent since AI has no face (maybe a robot's, at best).

In direct communications such as chats or patient interviews, AI has difficulty responding to outlier requests or questions that to the AI are vague or outside its algorithm's parameters.[54] We've all had the experience of conversing with a chatbot that doesn't understand our query. The risk can be for the AI to offer responses irrelevant to the question. AI doesn't have the awareness for the context of the query and so could offer answers that may be technically correct but unsuitable or even dangerous.[55] In one widely distributed example, when asked how to make cheese stick to pizza, AI replied "use non-toxic glue." Another example inquired about home remedies for appendicitis pain. AI's correct answer should've been for the person asking the question to call their doctor or seek immediate medical attention. However, AI suggested a high-fiber diet and an infusion of mint tea.

Long-term risks may arise because AI can "experience" hallucinations, whereby the machine-learning software powering the AI creates for itself an artificial world based on incorrect assumptions and biased data. And the longer the AI continues to cycle through this invented world, the more disconnected its responses are from reality.

---

53. Berkeley Public Health, "Can we replace human empathy in healthcare?" *Berkeley Public Health, Research Highlights*, June 11, 2021, https://publichealth.berkeley.edu/news-media/research-highlights/can-we-replace-human-empathy-in-healthcare.
54. Tom Greenhalgh, "How accurate is AI in customer support?" *Yuma*, July 11, 2024, https://yuma.ai/blogs/how-accurate-is-ai-in-customer-support.
55. Avram Piltch, "17 Cringe-worthy Google AI answers demonstrate the problem with training on the entire web," *Tom's Hardware, Tech Industry, Artificial Intelligence*, May 25, 2024, https://www.tomshardware.com/tech-industry/artificial-intelligence/cringe-worth-google-ai-overviews.

Reliance on AI in situations requiring bedside manner will erode patient confidence in their provider's healthcare, reinforcing an attitude that the physician and staff don't care for them, resulting in reduced adherence to treatment plans and a worsening of patient outcomes.

Remedies to prevent erroneous consequences from AI would be robust guardrails to prevent its replies from veering outside acceptable boundaries. One solution is when AI determines that it has reached its ability to provide acceptable and useful advice, it would hand off the exchange to a human.

The Sacred Covenant of Medicine

Let us remember that medicine is not merely a transactional exchange of services but a sacred covenant between healers and those seeking healing. In the pursuit of efficiency and financial success, we must not lose sight of the fact that every patient is a unique individual, deserving of care that extends beyond clinical procedures, and of an interaction dependent on and measured by bedside manner.

ACKNOWLEDGMENTS

I would like to extend my deepest gratitude to Edith Stillwagon, my high school chemistry teacher, whose passion for science ignited my curiosity and laid the groundwork for my dream of becoming a doctor. Your encouragement and belief in my potential have left a lasting impact on my life.

I am also profoundly thankful to Dr. Jonas, my cardiologist at Nassau County Medical Center, whose guidance and expertise not only shaped my medical career but also exemplified the compassion that defines our profession. Your dedication to your patients has been a beacon of inspiration.

To my incredible medical colleagues—thank you for your relentless commitment to making a difference in the lives of those who are sick or suffering. Your hard work and resilience are a testament to the healing power of medicine.

With heartfelt appreciation, I recognize the invaluable contributions of each of you in helping me achieve my dreams.

AUTHOR'S BIO

Dr. James Longobardi, a distinguished board-certified podiatrist, has dedicated over three decades to advancing foot and ankle care in San Diego, California. Born and raised on Long Island, New York, Dr. Longobardi's aspiration to become a doctor ignited at the tender age of eight. His journey began with a commitment to service in the United States Navy, where he served as a hospital corpsman with the United States Marine Corps at Quantico, Virginia.

Dr. Longobardi's medical career took flight after completing the physician's assistant program at George Washington University, where he excelled as a neurosurgery orthopedic shock trauma PA in the Washington, D.C. metropolitan area for seven years. His quest for further specialization led him to Des Moines, Iowa, where he pursued a degree in podiatry at Des Moines Medical College, College of Podiatry.

Following his education, Dr. Longobardi completed a rigorous surgical residency in San Diego, California. Over the past 34 years, he has been a pillar of the San Diego community, practicing in the Chula Vista suburb and specializing in limb salvage and forefoot reconstructive surgery. His expertise and dedication have earned him esteemed roles, including serving on the California Board of Podiatry and as the former Chief of Surgery at Scripps Mercy Chula Vista.

AUTHOR'S BIO

Dr. Longobardi's career reflects a profound commitment to advancing podiatric medicine and providing exceptional care, solidifying his reputation as a leading specialist in his field.

www.ingramcontent.com/pod-product-compliance
Lightning Source LLC
Chambersburg PA
CBHW071416220526
45469CB00004B/1297